SECRETS OF HEALTH AND FITNESS

MARK MEEK

outskirts
press

Outskirts Press, Inc.
http://www.outskirtspress.com

ISBN: 978-1-9772-1174-3

Outskirts Press and the "OP" logo are trademarks belonging to Outskirts Press, Inc.

PRINTED IN THE UNITED STATES OF AMERICA

Table of Contents

INTRODUCTION

When I was 15 years old, something just came over me and I got tired of feeling out of shape. I walked out to the porch and did five pushups. I have been a devout seeker of health and fitness from that day until now, more than 40 years later. This was a life-changing event, probably second only to finding God.

At age nearly 60 I have lived my life in near-perfect health. I have my hair and not much of it gray. My skin is about like it was when I was 20. I am doing daily workouts that I would have been very pleased with as a teenager. And this didn't come from my genes.

This book is about what I have learned. Fitness resolutions have a very high casualty rate. But there are differences between those that succeed and those that don't. Yours is going to be one of the ones that succeed. You have more control over your health and fitness than you probably ever realized.

Being in shape feels absolutely awesome. There is nothing that can replace it.

I am not going to tell you a bunch of stuff that you already know. If you have ever wondered if you should quit smoking or drinking alcohol or lose weight, the answer is "yes". This goes directly to what you have to do to revolutionize your health and fitness, and it is most definitely within your power. When you are finished with this book, you will not know everything but you will know what you need to know. You will see the path to your maximum potential for health and fitness.

I think anyone can get a lot of benefit from that is in this book, young or old, male or female. We usually think of strength training as being for men, but women can benefit greatly from a moderate amount of strength training, as well as for endurance and stamina. In days past, most women did work that required a significant amount of strength.

Please remember that exercise comes with some possibility of injury. Be careful and, depending on your present health, maybe check with your doctor first.

CHAPTER ONE

DIET

1) THE IMPORTANCE OF DIET

If you are an average person, you have practically no idea how important your diet is. The molecular bonds in foods contain energy. When the foods are digested, your body breaks some of the molecular bonds with stomach acid and uses the energy that is released for movement and bodily operations. The atoms and molecules are then used in building and repairing the body.

But not just any atoms and molecules will do for building the body. Your body is a very specialized machine, almost more specialized than we can comprehend. It needs certain atoms and molecules in certain amounts. If the body does not get the specific atoms and molecules that it needs it can synthesize molecules, at least to some extent, but that is a strain on the body and it is better if it doesn't have to. If the body does not have the atoms and molecules that it needs, not for energy but for building and repairing the body, it will, in most cases, still be able to operate but not as efficiently or for as long as if it did have what it needed.

That is where diet comes in. Our objective here is to make sure that your body always has just the right atoms and molecules that it needs for maximum efficiency.

The idea that our diet is very important is definitely not a fad. As time goes on, in news reports and research, it only gets more and more important. Fast food restaurants that were once synonomous with junk food now realize how much people want healthy food.

When I was young, sometimes I would be tired at work in ways that I am not now. The reason was that my diet had room for improvement. I always had a thing about push-ups, when I was a child I thought that being fit meant being able to do a lot of pushups. Even when I was mainly into weightlifting, I would still periodically test how many push-ups I could do. I got into the 70s many times but was never able to do 80. It wasn't until I was 45 years old that I finally got 80 and the reason is improvement in diet.

I used to read the exercise routines of various weightlifters and athletes in sports where strength is important. There would be the routines of both world-class athletes and "lo-cal" athletes at colleges and schools. What really stood out was diet. The more proficient the athlete was, the closer to world-class, the greater the relative importance of diet. A lot of the world-class athletes would actually start talking about their diets before their exercise routines. While the "local" athletes talked much more about exercise, many not mentioning diet at all.

What does that tell you about the vital importance of diet?

Most of us really don't need to be told what foods are good for you, and which aren't. But there is more to it than that. Getting a good diet isn't really complicated. But each person is different and getting just the right diet that is absolutely the best available for you takes some work, and that is what we are going to do here.

A person can study auto mechanics. But every make and model of car has it's own quirks. strengths and, weaknesses. Human bodies are the same way. What is good for someone else may not be as good, or may be better, for you.

I am a writer and much of what I write is about science. The place that I got my scientific way of thinking from is always looking for ways to improve my diet and exercise program, and I can tell you all that I have learned.

2) MODERN ADVANTAGES AND DISADVANTAGES CONCERNING DIET

Today, we are bombarded by information in the media about which foods are good for us. To most people, it is just common sense, although it would be nice if everyone agreed about which foods were good. But, on the other hand there are endless processed, and just plain junk, foods that are definitely not good. The reason that processed foods have become so popular is simply that they tend to be quick and convenient when most people are in a hurry.

The great disadvantage of modern life for health is that it is sedentary and requires far less physical work. It also has dietary disadvanatges in the production of inexpensive and easily available processed foods. By processed, I simply mean removed from the food's natural state. As a general rule, the further removed from nature a food is, the less healthy it is. It is sometimes said that "If you can pronounce the in-gredients then it's natural, if not then it's processed. But this is not a strict rule as many processed foods are specifically "fortified with vitamins and minerals", which is a good thing. Also remember that, when a given molecule enters your body, it does not matter if it is 'natural' or not, as long as it is the same molecule..

But the modern world also has great dietary advantages to offer. In times past, people certainly had a more wholesome diet. But that is true only if we consider the foods one-by-one. Each individual food may have been more wholesome but the diet lacked variety because, for the most part, the same few foods were being eaten at any given time of year. Before the developments of refrigeration, preservatives and rapid transportation, the only foods available was what was grown locally and in-season.

That is the primary reason why people in days past didn't live as long, on the average, as they do today. It was not that they didn't have nutritious foods, it was that they didn't have variety in those foods. Wheat and corn and apples and strawberries are all nutritious. But a diet of nothing but wheat and corn and apples and strawberries is not nutritious. They were getting nutrients but not all of the nutrients that they needed.

Supermarkets today are filled with foods from around the world. Instead of being stuck to the same few foods, at any given time of the year, we are now faced with an endless variety of foods. The downside is, as we might expect, that not all of those foods are nutritious.

Most of the world's population lives in the northern hemisphere so some nations in the southern hemisphere, like Chile in South America, have made the most of their location to ship all manner of produce while it is out-of-season in North America. And what we are going to do is to take advantage of the wide variety of foods that are available inexpensively to make sure that you get the best diet that you can get.

3) SUGAR AND SALT

Lets briefly discuss those two major perils of the modern diet, sugar and salt.

Sugar is addictive, both to the companies that manufacture

food products and to the consumers. Sugar is sweet and tasty. One great advantage of sugar is that if energy is required as soon as possible, nothing is better than sugar. The energy of sugary foods like chocolate become available to the body very quickly.

As far as producing sweet foods, it often doesn't even have to be sugar. Corn starch is very widely used and it is inexpensive and relatively easy for manufacturers to work with.

Sugary foods are often described as "empty calories". As described above we use food first for the energy in the molecular bonds, and then use the atoms and molecules as building blocks after the energy has been released. "Empty calories" means that the food contains energy, but doesn't leave the body much in the way of valuable atoms and molecules. Since calories are generally much more easily available than the nutritional atoms and molecules that we need, we should be trying to get the best nutritional value for the calories that we take in and "empty calories" means that we are not getting much of such value.

Sugar not only causes excessive weight gain, albeit poor nutrition, it also decays the teeth.

Humans require salt, but only a little bit. Like sugar, salt is inexpensive and addictive to both consumers and manufacturers.

For consumers, salt is tasty. For manufacturers, salt is an effective and convenient natural preservative. A food that contains salt will have a longer shelf life than one that doesn't, and that increases the chances that the food will be sold before it has to be discarded.

The trouble with salt is that it causes water retention. This can bring about all kinds of health issues. For one thing, it means making the heart work harder to pump blood.

4) THE GOODNESS OF FOODS REMOVED

Manufacturers of food products often purposely take the nutritious part out, leaving foods that tend to be white in color. Wheat is highly nutritious, it acts as "roughage" to clean out the system and prevent maladies such as colon cancer. But some people, particularly the elderly, cannot digest wheat. In a family gathering, there is a significant chance that someone there will be unable to digest wheat.

So what manufacturers of wheat-based products like bread and pasta do is to simply remove it, leaving white bread and white pasta. The trouble is that the part they are removing is the nutritious part. Bread and pasta should always be whole-wheat. There is oat bread for those who cannot digest wheat. Oat is, if anything, more nutritious than wheat.

The same principle applies to sugar. "Real" sugar, whether from cane or beet, is nothing like as damaging as the processed and refined white version of the sugar that most people buy.

The other food that gets the goodness taken out of it is rice. Rice is far and away the most common food in the world as a whole, no other food comes remotely close. But white rice has had the goodness taken out of it to make it easier to digest. Long-grain rice is the good one.

5) BASIC PRINCIPLES OF YOUR DIET

Let's get on with the basic principles of your diet. These are the things that you will be having every day, or will have at every opportunity.

The first and foremost almost goes without saying. Drink an abundance of water every day. You are made mostly of water. Your body is something like 75% water. Of course you have to have plenty of water to be in good health. I just drink tap water but if you want to pay for bottled water, that's fine. I have a large bottle that I fill with water every day. The body can conserve water when it doesn't have enough, but that is a strain on the body and there is no reason for it to not have enough.

Most people eat before they are hungry but wait until they are thirsty to drink. What you should do is exactly the opposite. Drink water even when you don't feel thirsty. Even if your body doesn't need the water it will help to clean out your system.

Always have a generous helping of green leafy vegetables at least once a day. I usually have spinach or kale but it must be fresh and green and leafy. This is the most common-sense dietary rule that there is.

All fruit and vegetables are good. But some really stand out. Berries may cost money but try to have some at every opportunity. Raspberries, blackberries, blueberries and, cranberries are extremely beneficial. If cancer cells could think, berries and cherries would be their worst nightmare.

Another thing that I have every day is tomato. I rarely have a whole tomato, usually sun-dried or pre-diced tomato that they sell at my local supermarket.

If losing weight is not a concern, make sure to have a variety of nuts and sunflower seeds every day. But they do have calories so hold off if weight loss is an important part of your plan.

I am not into supplements. I am not saying that they are bad, just that I do not take them myself. The only one that I take sometimes is omega-3 fish oil, and I take that to help my brain to think.

But what I am a great believer in is spices. Spices are generally inexpensive and they add flavor to a meal. Most importantly, they get valuable atoms and molecules into your body that you probably wouldn't get otherwise. Possibly the primary reason that Europeans set about exploring the world centuries ago was to find sources of spices that they couldn't get at home. But today, you have a wide variety of spices from all over the world available in virtually any supermarket. I see that as a great opportunity to take advantage of. There is a list of the spices that I use below.

These are going to be your "everyday" foods.

6) THE WONDER OF CARROTS

I am always looking to see how I can improve in the area of health and fitness. But let me tell you about one mistake that I made. I decided that I could do without carrots, that I was getting the nutrients that I need without them.

As the saying goes, "Everybody makes mistakes".

I went about eight months without carrots before realizing what a mistake it was. The reason that I started going without carrots is that I tried a new nutrition bar and it seemed like my vision was improving, leading me to believe that I didn't need carrots any more.

But my vision eventually started to suffer, and I presumed that it was just due to my eyes gradually "getting old". One day I went to read the Sunday newspaper and I really struggled to read it. My eyes were really taking their time focusing on the words. It took me longer to read the newspaper than it usually does.

My eyes started to "look old". It didn't seem to affect the rest of my body that much, at least as I could tell, but my eyes really began to deteriorate after a few months without carrots.

But then I realized my mistake. I am back to my "carrots everyday" rule. My eyes are thoroughly grateful. I can read the newspaper easily without glasses even in relatively dim light. My eyes do not "look old", not at all.

Nobody except Bugs Bunny will say that carrots are their favorite food. I find them to be rather tasteless. But I have learned my lesson and carrots are my wonder food. If I had to choose my number one food, this would be it. Ironically, it's brightly colored fruits and vegetables that are good for the eyes.

Do women know that it's virtually impossible to eat vegetables often, and carrots in particular, without being attractive?

I get canned carrots, which are inexpensive and available everywhere. Raw carrots might be perilous for the teeth. Make sure to have a generous helping, not just a few small slices of carrot.

I would like to get a picture of Bugs Bunny with a carrot to put on my wall. Carrots are awesome.

7) YOUR HAIR

I do not think that a man's hair, or lack of it, has anything whatsoever to do with his health and fitness. I also think that gray hair on a woman can look as good as any other color.

But hair can be important psychologically. Fortunately, there is an effective diet for your hair and it's good for the rest of your body too. That is one thing that we have going for us when it comes to diet. Something that is good for one part of your body, or aspect of your health, tends to be good for your whole body and your health in general. It would get really complicated if something were good for one part of your body but bad for another.

Attitudes to baldness vary with culture. Have you ever noticed that the U.S. has never had a bald president? But I think every man would at least like to have the option to keep his hair, and get a lot of it back if it has been lost.

There is an effective natural solution, and it is avacados. If you don't like avocado fruit, and a lot of people don't, then use avocado oil just as you would use olive oil. Avocado oil isn't really any more expensive than olive oil and it is very nutritious. Be generous with it and use it as you would olive oil. There should be a store with it.

What about gray hair? There is a simple solution to that too. Chickpeas (or garbanzos) literally remove the gray from hair. As with avocados, if you don't like chickpeas there is pasta available that it made from chickpeas. I have that twice a week and have only a little bit of gray in my hair.

For generally good hair, there is lentils. I find lentils to be very good overall and thay are a kind of a "foundation" of my diet, which I will get to shortly. Lentils are not only good for the hair, but for the whole body. Did you know that when lenses were invented, they were called "lenses" because they were shaped like lentils?

8) WEEKLY DIET CYCLING

As we have seen, people had wholesome foods in the past but their diets lacked variety. At any particualr time of year, they were having the same few foods over and over. A variety of healthy foods is very important. No one food or six foods have all that you need.

There are many different foods in your local supermarket, especially the fruits and vegetables, that would be healthy and nutritious. The more variety you could get the more likely the better. But you couldn't eat or afford all that is healthy. So what do you do?

The solution is to cycle foods by the week, as most people do their grocery shopping by the week. You will get some of the same foods every week, we'll call these your "staples". But to get the healthiest variety, you will cycle the others.

Let's start with fruit. You should have at least two different fruits per week, a serving of each every day. One week it might be apples and bananas, the next week it might be kiwis and plums. Then a month later, or you could try six-week cycling maybe with each fruit twice, you would come back to apples and bananas. It does, of course, depend on what's available.

Remember the old saying "An apple a day keeps the doctor away". Apples also have the advatage of cleaning the teeth. An apple as the last food of the day will be good for the teeth.

You will be having a generous portion of leafy fresh green vegetables every day. But one week you might get spinach, the next week kale, and the following week some kind of leafy green mix.

Your bread should always be whole grain, whole wheat or, oat, never white, but you can vary the exact bread by the week.

Berries and cherries, cancer's worst enemies, are very nutritious but sometimes expensive and seasonal. You can vary tham by the week, if necessary, one week blueberries, one week blackberries, one week raspberries and, one week cherries. But if they are available and affordable enough to have all the time, that is even better. Berries are another "wonder food".

The healthiest diet has not only healthy foods but a variety of healthy foods. Fortunately, it is not necessary to have every healthy food because some contain the same beneficial nutrients.

9) THE MAIN MEAL

Let me describe what I call my "Main Meal". This is just how I do it, not to say you have to do it the same way. But this works for me in "putting everything together".

My main meal is a mix. I start with lentils and then mix other things in. Except for my green leafy vegetable and carrots, which I have on the side.

The lentils are constant, long-grain rice can also be used, but everything else is variable. That is how I get variety by the week.

My lentil mix is different all the time. Some days diced onion gets mixed in. Almost always olives, sometimes black olives and sometimes green. I mix in capers and raisins, prunes or, sliced dates. Sometimes corn and sometimes peas. Sliced mushrooms usually daily.

Tomatoes are a daily staple so if I don't have sun-dried tomatoes on the side, I will mix in diced tomatoes.

This is one way that I accomodate variety, starting with lentils and then mixing other nutritious things in, with the mix varying all the time.

Such a mix serves another purpose. It is the place to put my spices. Spices are sold in powder form and I sprinkle them onto the mix. Then I wash the spices into the mix with my daily avocado oil, as described above. I usually top that off with something tasty, like Worcestershire Sauce which is also spicy.

So there it is. With this mix concept I can accomodate the necessary variety of food, have a place to put my ration of spices, and get my quota of avocado oil. I usually have this mix five days a week and the pasta made from chickpeas, as described above, the other two days. But the leafy green vegetables, carrots and tomatoes every day.

10) THE ACID STRATEGY

There is a diet strategy that I have developed that I think every "older" person should practice. It doesn't involve any "new" foods but is a digestion strategy.

We know that the body, in general, tends to get less efficient as we age. We try to counteract that aging with diet and exercise.

Now here is the question. If the body in general gets less efficient with age, then what about the digestive system? That should also be getting less efficient.

We try to counteract aging with diet and exercise. But the only way to exercise the digestive system is to eat, which we do anyway. This must mean that if we are on a good balanced diet as we age, our diet is effectively deteriorating not because of the nature of the diet but because of the declining efficiency of our digestive system. The quality of our diet is effectively declining not because of the quality of the diet but because of our ability to effectively digest it.

We can refer to the nutrients that are actually digested into the body as the "Digested Diet". It is different from our actual diet because it depends on the efficiency of our digestive system. Our diet naturally gets poorer as we age, even if we are eating the same good diet, and this is a primary reason behind aging.

Studies about diet tend to presume that the digestive system is 100% efficient, which it isn't.

So what can be done about it? What if there was a food that was nutritious for the digestive system itself? Or some way to improve the digestive system, rather than just the diet?

The digestive system operates on acid, the stomach acid that breaks foods down. When we age the efficiency of that process should naturally decrease, so that the effective quality of our diet also decreases. But what if we could give the stomach a little bit more acid, especially at meal times? I got this idea because I sometimes felt that my digestion process was less than 100% efficient.

What I do now is to have a relatively small amount of Coca-Cola after a meal. I drink Coke Zero, which has no calories. It seems to me to work very well, I have followed this procedure for years and do not feel any indigestion. That means that my body, and digestive system, is getting near the full available notritional value of the food.

There is one thing that has to be kept in mind. Part of your diet is to drink a lot of water. But do not drink a lot of liquid right at mealtime. While the water will help to move the food along in the digestive system, it won't help to break the food down because that requires acid, and it will dilute the acid that you do take in to assist with digestion.

I use Coke Zero, mainly because I like it even though it is not considered as a nutritious food. You can get acid from whatever source you like, maybe an orange with every meal. The obvious source of acid is citrus, maybe the juice of a lemon. We are always told to eat a nutritious diet but no one ever seems to mention the efficiency of the digestive system and how it should decline with age. To get a really nutritious diet we have to counteract that inefficiency. That is one of the cornerstones of my diet.

11) NUTRITIONAL WORDS

It is impossible for me to make a list of everything that is good for you, and that isn't what I want to do with this book anyway. The method that I am going to use is nutritional words. These are the kinds of words that you should be looking for when you buy foods. Beware of the simple words "wheat flour", all flour is wheat flour. What you want to avoid is white breads with the goodness removed.

Oat
Bran
Whole Wheat

Whole Grain
Multigrain
Fiber
Antioxidants
Roughage
Vitamins
Protein

SPICES

After careful study, here are the spices that I decided on as a part of my daily diet. Spices are generally inexpensive and get valuable molecules into your body that you would likely not get otherwise. Not using spices really doesn't make sense.

Curry is the mix of spices that smells like an Indian restaurant. Indians have been perfecting the mix for hundreds of years. They generally serve it as a sauce but you can just buy the powder.

Tumeric is supposed to be absolutely wonderful for general health. But sometimes the body has difficulty absorbing it so you should use ordinary pepper with it, which is the world's most common spice. I know there is some skepticism about "wonder" spices, but enough people are convinced so there is probably something good about it. Anyway, it's flavorful and not expensive.

Ginger has been so highly prized for so long that there must be something good about it.

The same can be said for cinnamon, which has been highly valued since far back into ancient times. It is not just a flavoring, it is supposed to be very good for health. They used to have to get it from the other side of the world. Now you can get it from the local supermarket.

Some kind of peppers. I use red pepper and chili powder.

Basil Leaves.

Garlic is another one that has been highly prized far back into ancient times. There just has to be something good about it.

My local supermarket used to have "The Chinese Five" spice, and I used to get it, but they don't carry it anymore.

The spice trade between different parts of the world is a highly fabled and legendary part of human history. Many famous explorers were looking for spices as much as for gold. Even ordinary pepper used to be highly valued in the west at one time. Just be glad that today you have all of these spices easily and inexpensively available at your local supermarket.

NUTRITION BARS

Quite a bit of my diet consists of nutrition bars. They are easy, convenient, usually inexpensive, and generally nutritious. I get ones made of oat, which is highly nutritious. You can research any particular ones online. Nutrition bars are designed to combine quick energy with good nutrition. If you are weight-conscious, and plan to have a nutrition bar for dessert, but then want something before mealtime, nutrition bars are conventient in that you can have it now and it will give you energy, instead of for dessert later.

DRINKS

I don't drink alcohol at all but there are always articles about the health benefits of one glass of wine. People in France have quite a bit of fat in their diet, being particularly fond of cheese. But yet they have a low rate of heart disease that is commonly credited to wine, which supposedly stops plaque from building up in the arteries.

What I have always drank a lot of is tea. I just have black tea but green tea is supposed to be even better. It is believed to be healthy and I certainly believe that it is.

However, as stated above, your main drink should be water. It is a good idea to have a large bottle and fill it every day. I just drink tap water but you can pay for bottled water if you want to. Give your body even more water than it needs, we are mostly made of water. Most people eat before they are hungry, but wait until they are thirsty to drink. What you should do is just the opposite.

So your next trip to the supermarket will be the beginning of your new diet. If you are an average person, it will be one of the best changes you have ever made.

EXERCISE

1) BENEFITS OF EXERCISE

Diet alone cannot get you to the best possible health and fitness. You must also exercise.

Why do you suppose that so many people struggle in gyms? Because it is worth it, that's why. The benefits of a sensible exercise program are incalculable. If anyone ever came up with a pill that could provide all of the benefits of exercise, it would be the greatest invention that the world has ever seen. Being fit and strong and healthy feels just awesome, and there is no replacement for it. I have never heard of anyone regretting undertaking an exercise program.

Once you get into an appropriate exercise program you will want to do more. It is addictive, but a positive kind of addiction. Runners refer to the "runner's high". Weightlifters call it "being bitten by the iron bug".

One day, when I was 15 years old, something just came over me and I got fed up with feeling out-of-shape. I decided that something had to be done about it and I walked out to the porch and did five pushups. More than forty years have passed since that day, and I have been a devout exerciser ever since. I have also been learning all of that time and that is what I want to share here in this book.

The lessons of exercise carry over into other things in life. I have gained a strong sense of improvement. The motto of the U.S. state where I live is "Excelsior", which means "ever-upward". Just take wherever you are, whatever you can do, and just keep improving on it. That attitude will stay with you beyond exercise.

I learned that from exercising. A sense of continuous improvement comes from always trying to improve your own records or times in exercises. Just the feeling that with a smart application of effort things can be made better.

Much of the writing that I do is about science. I have been interested in science since childhood but I really got my scientific way of thinking from exercise. My gym was a laboratory where I was always looking for a better or more efficient exercise program, or a way to get more out of it. That has carried over to my scientific writing.

Everyone has their own exercise goals and some of what I

write here may not apply to you, at least not yet. But you may talk to other people who exercise and it wouldn't be a bad idea to "learn the lingo". You may also find lessons that can apply to the way that you are going to exercise.

2) PHYSIOLOGY

Lets have a look at what fitness means and how exercise works with the body.

There are several components of fitness. I would break it down into five. These are 1) strength 2) stamina 3) endurance 4) flexibility 5) motor skills.

Strength is how much effort your muscles can put into a task, such as lifting a weight. Endurance is how long your muscles can keep up that effort for. Stamina is how long your cardiovascular system, your heart and lungs, can support the effort. Flexibility is how maneuverable your body is, the most common flexibility exercise is touching your toes. Motor skills are movements particular to a certain sport or activity that are so well-practiced as to be "second nature" to your body.

Take note of the difference between endurance and stamina. The two often get considered together but are two distinct aspects. Endurance refers to how long the muscles can sustain an effort while stamina refers to how long the cardiovascular system can sustain the effort.

If a muscular effort is near one's capacity for exerting that effort, such as lifting something heavy, then the effort is a test of strength.

In a repetitive or continuous effort if strength is not much of a factor in the beginning or the first repetirion of the exercise then how many times, or for how long, the effort can be continued is a test of endurance. A common endurance exercise for the muscles of the upper body is how many pushups someone can do. But if that person could only do a very few pushups then it would be more a test of strength.

If neither strength nor endurance is the limiting factor in a repetitive or continuous effort then how long it can be sustained for is a test of stamina. Remember that stamina refers to the cardiovascular system while endurance refers to the muscles. The classic test of stamina is running. A person is strong enough to run, and the muscles of the legs have enough endurance, but the limiting factor is how long the heart and lungs can keep supplying the necessary oxygen.

If the limiting factor is whether or not the muscles are capable of exerting the necessary effort, for one or a few repetitions of the effort, then it is a test of strength.

If the limiting factor is not strength but how long the muscles can keep up the effort, then it is a test of endurance.

If the limiting factor is not strength or how long the muscles can keep up the effort, but for how long the heart and lung system can supply the necessary oxygen, then it is a test of stamina.

Strength is commonly tested by how much weight someone can lift, endurance by how many pushups or pull-ups they can do, and stamina by how far they can run. Another way that stamina can be measured is by pulse rate relative to activity. If a person has a lower pulse rate after doing the same activity that they did before, then their stamina is improving because the heart is working less to supply the necessary oxygen. Activity causes the muscles to increase their demand for oxygen.

When skeletal (voluntary) muscles are used, it causes a buildup of lactic acid. This is continuously generated by the muscles, but then removed. But when it is generated faster than it is being removed, it limits how long the muscles can be used for. This is known as endurance.

Strength is built mainly by enlarging and improving the muscles. Building endurance and stamina is by chemical changes. All three are "high-energy" states that must be maintained or they will deteriorate. That is why it is easier to get out of shape than to get into shape. But the muscles and the body seem to have a "memory" with regard to fitness. Once you have been in shape, it is generally easier to get back into shape than it would be if you had never been in shape.

Strength tends to last the longest. If a person has all-around fitness, strength, endurance and, stamina, and then suddenly becomes inactive so that the fitness gradually deteriorates, stamina will deteriorate fastest, endurance next, and strength will last the longest.

We have to be careful when comparing one person to another with regard to strength, endurance and, stamina. Body type is a factor also. With other factors being equal, if two people lift a given weight in the same way, a shorter person would have an innate advantage simply because they do not have to lift the weight as far. If two people undergo a test of stamina, such as pushups or pull-ups (chin-ups), the person who weighs less will have an advanatge because they are not lifting as much weight with each repetition of the exercise. If two people undergo a test of stamina, such as how far they can run, the taller person will have an advantage since they can move further per step.

There are three different types of muscle tissue. These are voluntary (or skeletal), involuntary and, cardiac muscles. The muscles that we can use when we choose are the voluntary, or skeletal, muscles. These muscles are attached to the bones, so that they can move the body, by tendons and ligaments, and the bones benefit from exercise too. Involuntary muscles are those used in such processes as breathing and digestion. Cardiac muscle is very special in that endurance is not a factor. That is why your heart can keep beating for your entire life.

All physical movements that are driven by voluntary use of

the skeletal muscles are either pushing or pulling motions. But muscles themselves can only contract when they are used. That is why muscles tend to operate in pairs, when one contracts the other relaxes. An obcious example is the biceps and triceps of the upper arms. The development of motor skills, specific to any sport or activity, is to train the active muscle to completely contract, while the opposing muscle in the pair completely relaxes.

Even when the skeletal (voluntary) muscles are not being used, they are held taut with a certain amount of tension. This is known as "tone". Well-toned muscles are a sign of physical fitness.

Muscle tissue weighs more than fat. This means that you can actually be gaining weight even though you are getting into shape and losing fat.

The way that exercise works is that it actually tears the muscle down. But then your body builds the muscle back up again. To adapt to the demand being placed on it, the body builds the muscle a little bit stronger than it was before. That is the principle of exercise, the muscles gradually get stronger because they are building back up after being broken down by exercise.

This means that the muscles need rest in order to grow. Your muscles actually grow and strengthen when you are resting and sleeping, not while you are exercising. If you exercise and the muscles are sore the next day, that is their way of telling you that the exercise is working and they need more recovery time before being used again. When you exercise and then are hungrier than usual the next day, that also means that the exercise is working and your body is asking for more protein and nutrinets so that it can build the muscles back up.

It would be good to familiarize yourself with the general muscle groups of the body. The neck muscles move the head. The biceps pull the forearm toward it, the opposing triceps straighten the arm. The muscles of the forearms control the hands. The deltoid muscles, at the ends of the shoulders, raise the arms. The pectoral muscles pull the arms across the chest. The back muscles pull the arms in the opposite direction, in order to lift something. The thigh muscles operate the legs. The calf muscles operate the feet in a way similar to how the forearm muscles operate the hands.

Each exercise movement has a "top" and a "bottom". Moving from bottom to top is the positive side of the exercise. Moving from top back down to bottom is the negative side. It is generally the positive side that works against gravity, making that the productive side. The maximum or "max" of an exercise is simply going all-out to lift as much, run as far, or doing as many repetitions of an exercise that you can do.

3) SKILL

Don't forget that an important part of any muscular

movement, including any exercise, is the skill involved in doing it. The motor skills, which I consider as one of the five components of fitness as described above, is the movements involved in any activity or sport that are so well-practiced that they become innate or second-nature.

What this means is that a major part of being able to lift something is knowing the most efficient way to lift it. In any lifting or moving motion, the body is a complex system of levers and there is a specific way to accomplish any physical task that is at the peak of efficiency.

In the same way, an important part of stamina is knowing how to pace oneself. To undertake a long run or marathon, the thing to do is not to start off as fast as possible. It is to pace oneself so that too much time is not lost in the beginning but yet the runner "leaves something for the finish".

Athletic or exercise performance is not just working hard but "working smart". But this is why we should not expect progress in an exercise program to continue at as rapid of a pace as at the beginning. Much of the iniitial progress in the program is due to the mastering of the motor skills of the exercises, rather than strength, endurance or, stamina. Once the motor skills of the movements are mastered by the body, there is no more progress in that direction and the rate of gain inevitably slows down.

4) BASIC PRINCIPLES OF YOUR EXERCISE PROGRAM

EXERCISE THE ENTIRE BODY THROUGH FULL RANGE OF MOTION

You must exercise the entire body. This is vitally important. The body is a very coordinated system. If you exercise only some parts of the body, you will never make as much progress as you would if you exercised the entire body. If the development of the body is uneven, the body "knows" about it and the undeveloped parts hold back the others.

Some lines of work provide exercise for the body but I have never seen any work that exercises the entire body roughly equally. This makes an organized exercise program indispensible.

When exercising, the muscles involved must be taken through their full range of motion. Isometric and isotonic exercises used to be popular as being easy to do anywhere during the course of the day. Isometric is pitting two muscle groups against each other and isotonic is putting a muscular effort against a stationary object.

I have found it difficult to get the best results from these exercises and the reason is simple. They do not take the muscles through their full range of motion. Muscles must be exercised as they are made to be used. This necessarily involves not only the effort of those muscles but also effort through the full range of their motion.

Exercise devices are another option but many do not take the muscles through their full range of motion.

VARY THE EXERCISE PROGRAM

Have you ever seen two people who begin exercising at about the same time, they seem about equally capable and motivated and make progress at about the same rate. But then one seems to continue making progress while the other slows down, and you wonder why.

The answer may be diet, which is a lot more important than the average person apparently thinks it is. But if both have a diet of fairly equal quality then there is one more thing that it might be, and it is something that is very important to understand about exercise.

This other factor is variation. If you do your exercises in the same way all the time, while it is certainly better than not doing anything, your body will adapt to the demand and then your progress will level off. To keep making progress, it is necessary to work the muscles in different ways and from different angles. Along with diet, this is often what makes the difference between making progress and not making progress.

Switch up your exercise program periodically. When you do the same exercises you can put variety into them, hitting the muscles from different angles, by varying the distance between your hands, when doing exercises like pushups or pull-ups, and changing the positioning of your feet a little bit when doing exercises like knee bends. Even something as simple as this will help to work the muscles from different angles and keep your progress going.

I have two different workouts but I alternate them, on different days, to provide variety. Many athletes in seasonal sports alternate by season, training for stamina and practicing the sport itself during the season and doing strength training in the off-season. Many athletes who train with weights for a particular sport have gotten more interested in the weights than in the sport itself.

Training for a sport might also alternate days, practicing the sport itself on one day and then doing exercises on alternate days. When training in the same way all the time, the Law of Diminishing Returns will set in. The way to keep it away, and to keep making progress, is variety. Periodically vary the exercises and continuously vary, even if slightly, the angle at which the exercise works the muscles.

Let me just mention one thing that I notice about weight training. When I would read the exercise routines of athletes in spotrs where strength is important, sometimes "world class" athletes, and sometimes "local" athletes, I noticed something interesting. Barbells are weights that are held with two hands, and dumbells with one hand. I notice that "world class" athletes tend to make more use of dumbells, relative to barbells, than "local" athletes.

Clearly, there is some kind of benefit involved with using dumbells for at least some of the workout. The reason is variation. A weight in each hand offers more potential difference in the angles at which the muscles can be worked than a barbell held with one hand. There is a lesson in that for any exercise on the benefit of variation to keep The Law of Diminishing Returns at bay.

INJURY PREVENTION

Another fundamental principle of a successful exercise program is injury prevention. Obviously, you cannot make progress in exercise if you sustain an injury.

Part of injury prevention will come with learning the motor skills of the movements. A smooth, even motion is the way to avoid injury.

Another part of injury prevention is evenly developing the muscle groups of the body. The muscles work together in different movements and having one more developed then another invites injury to the weaker muscle.

But probably the most immediate measure to prevent injury is warming up and stretching the muscles just prior to exercise. It also may be better to exercise where it is warm. It is much easier to injure a muscle when the muscle is cold. Warming up can be simple, touching the toes and swinging the arms back and forth a few times, getting more blood flowing in the muscles, before proceeding with exercise.

It also may help to speed progress, and avoid injury, to exercise when your body is "expecting" it, meaning at around the same time every day.

Soreness in the muscles the next day after a workout means that the exercise is working. You have succeeded in the "breaking down" phase of the exercise and your body is asking for a little bit more time to build the muscle back up before you use it again. But soreness will be mostly eliminated by steady exercise and experience. You will know just the right amount of exercise to do that will not be too much. Soreness also comes when you exercise again after missing it, or do an exercise that you haven't done in a while, or haven't previously done at all, because it is working the muscles in a new way.

So the basic principles of your exercise program are going to be: 1) Development of the entire body. 2) Taking the muscles through their full range of motion. 3) Vary the exercises and work the muscles from different angles and, 4) Prevent injuries that halt progress.

5) TIME

HOW MUCH TIME CAN YOU PUT INTO EXERCISE?

Here is a question that everyone who has a successful exercise program has an answer to. The question is not even about exercise or fitness, it is about your life. This simple question is as important as anything in determining whether you can get fit.

The question is as follows: How much time can you realistically put into this?

That is all-important. How much time? Also what time of day will you do your exercises? Can you sacrifice a television program and do it then?

If you get on an exercise program that takes too much time, you will likely just end up not doing it at all. Many people who want to get fit ask an athlete who they know to draw up an exercise program for them. The trouble is that it is too ambitious, or takes too much time, or they are not able to do it, or it doesn't really fit with what they want from exercise, and they end up just not doing it at all.

Even if you are really enthusiastic about exercising, which is great, do not underestimate how important time is. Time is what life is made of and if your exercise routing takes up more of it than you are really able to give, then it will not last. It is better to have a somewhat lesser program that at least you are really going to do than to have a more ambitious program that you are not going to do for long.

Sometimes unexpected things happen so that we do not have enough time to exercise. If life always went according to schedule that would be wonderful, but it doesn't. What I used to do is have a long workout and a short workout. I would try to do the long one, but if I just couldn't then I would do the short one. if I didn't have time for either one, I would just do three exercise sets, a set of pushups for the upper body, twists for the midsection and, knee bends for the legs.

Today I exercise four days a week on weekdays, usually missing Friday but I can make up a workout then if I have missed one. If that is not possible, I will just do those basic three sets instead of a full workout. In our hurried world, it is adaptability and time management like this that makes all the difference in keeping an exercise program going.

It is true that exercise takes time. But it somewhat "pays for itself" in that you handle sleep more efficiently when you are fit, and so do not need quite as much of it. If you wanted to you could get up earlier and exercise.

HOME OR GYM

Here is another question, although it doesn't have to be answered just yet. Are you going to exercise at home or go to a gym?

There are great advantages to going to a gym. The equipment. Being around other people that are exercising, and maybe benefitting from their knowledge and enthusiasm. If the gym is staffed, there may be trainers to help, encourage and, advise you.

I used to be a regular at the local gym. But I haven't been there in years. There is a reason that I stopped going, and that reason is time.

I am not necessarily saying that this will apply to you. But what I took into account is that it took 15 or 20 minutes to drive to the gym each way, plus getting changed. I certainly did not have all of the equipment at home that they had at the gym. But exercising at home gave me more of that all-important factor known as time. I went to the gym when I was young and still learning, and where someone could spot me on a heavy bench press, but in the long term I got more done by exercising at home because it gave me more time to exercise.

There used to be a controversy about which was better, a Universal Gym which had weights in stacks, or free weights. Virtually everyone agreed that free weights were superior to a Universal Gym for results.

But not so fast, there was more to it than that. With free weights, it was necessary to change the weight whenever a different amount of weight was required on the bar, and that took time. With the Universal Gym, all that was necessary to change the weight was to put the pin in another slot. If a person only had a limited amount of time to exercise, they could get more done on the Universal Gym than with free weights and, for many people, that was enough to offset the quality superiority of free weights.

By the way, the reason that free weights were generally considered as superior to the Universal Gym, at least if an equal amount of exercise was being done, is that the movement of free weights has more potential for variety, as we saw above, because in a Universal Gym the weight moves in one straight line on a rack.

You should have a workout period. But that doesn't necessarily mean that all of your exercise has to be done in one session. There can be other exercises that you do at odd times during the day.

6) LIFECYCLES AND CHANGES

Another potential workout peril is moving. You often hear someone say something like "I was always going to the gym where I used to live. But after moving, I just got away from it. There wasn't a gym near where I lived like there was before. I used to know everybody at the gym. I lived in a house but now I am in an apartment and that makes working out at home more difficult. I don't want to exercise knowing that people are in the apartment below me and it might make noise. The grocery store where I now shop doesn't seem to have the same nutritious foods that I used to buy, or at least not where I can see them. So, I just haven't been exercising since moving here".

But that is where your resourcefulness and adaptation comes in. There is a way to continue exercising, and to keep making progress, in your new home, you just have to find it. Look online for ideas to see how others have exercised in an apartment, where there probably wouldn't be a place and you wouldn't be able to use much exercise equipment. When I lived in an apartment I thought of this and asked for one on the ground floor.

If you age and are not able to do some of the training that you used to, the same improvising and adaptation applies. Just make an exercise program of whatever you can do. If I was 90 years old and the only exercise I could do was to move my arms around, then you can be sure that I will make an exercise routine out of that. What I find about age is not that I can't exercise, it's that I can't "get away" with things like I could when I was younger. I have to do things "just right". This means keeping up a good diet and not missing many workouts.

Lifecycle changes inevitably affect your exercise program. Suppose that you are a young athlete who makes physical training a priority. What happens years later if you have a family and career? There is a good chance that it will mean the end of most of your physical training.

My lifecycle plan was to do calisthenics, such as pushups, pull-ups and, knee bends as a teenager. After high school I got into weight lifting, which I continued for a number of years. In my thirties, I got back into the calisthenics that I had done earlier. In my opinion lifting heavy weights before the spine is fully grown, at about age 17, can make a person shorter than they would have been otherwise. When I got back into calisthenics, it maintained most of the reserve of strength that I had built up by weightlifting. But the calisthenics took less time and were more portable and today, at nearly age 60, I have lived my life in nearly perfect health and am doing daily workouts that I would have been very pleased with as a teenager.

7) DEFINITION

Next, we come to another important question. Clearly you want to be fit. But what exactly does that mean to you? Fitness can mean many different things. Health, basically freedom from disease and ailments, is actually much simpler to define than physical fitness.

Suppose someone said that they wanted to be educated. You would probably wonder what exactly they meant by it. Being "educated" can mean many things. Most people that are educated have one or two fields of study that they have concentrated on, and a broad general set of knowledge beyond that. What will be the focus of their education? Will it be medicine? Or science? Or history?

The same concept applies to physical fitness. It is good to be fit, as it is to be educated. But, as with education, fitness can mean many different things.

Before going any further stop and think about exactly what fitness means to you. This is so important because fitness programs have a high casualty rate and people who continue a successful fitness program tend to have a strong definition of what exactly fitness means to them.

Do you want to be strong? Do you want to be a runner? Do you want to be fit to play a particular sport? Are you recovering from being hospitalized? Do you know people who play tennis and want to play too? Do you want to lose weight and have more energy and look better? Is Father

Time closing in on you and you want to strike back?

When people go to college, they choose what they want to major in according to what fits their interests and aptitudes. This certainly gets better results than having the government tell students what to major in. Sometimes students change their majors. How successful a student is depends on how interested they are in the subject.

Exactly the same concept applies to a fitness program. The trouble with an exercise program that someone else has drawn up for you is that it may not be a perfect fit for either your interests or your aptitudes or your time factor. Most people know someone who is really into working out who can draw up a program for them, or can get a program online. But athletes tend to think that everybody should be like them, and the program may well not be one that the person is going to keep up with for long.

Having someone draw up an exercise program for you is a lot like asking someone what you should major in at college. It is a lot better if you choose what you want to do, although you may change that choice at a later time. The fitness program that you are most likely to continue is the one you develop yourself.

Training for a sport is relatively straightforward but seeking general "fitness" is more nebulous. For a program that you are actually going to continue doing, it needs to be defined, even if you may decide to change the definition at some point in the future.

So, starting now, spend some time thinking about exactly what physical fitness means to you. What do you want to do with your fitness? What do want to look like or be able to do that you can't do now? It may be an interim goal on your way to an ultimate goal. People who have a successful exercise program tend to be the ones who have a clear answer to this question.

8) WEIGHT LOSS

Weight loss is at least part of the goal of some, perhaps even the majority, of people who begin an exercise program. Our bodies are designed to be physically active, and to eat natural foods. Because food might not always be readily available, our bodies are designed to be able to store energy as fat so that we can survive in the meantime. But modern technology has made it not only so that physical exertion is far less necessary than it used to be but that a wide variey of processed, and just plain junk, foods are available to us, and we have yet to adapt.

If I had to define our era in a single sentence, my definition would be "We have reached the point where we can change the world faster than we can adapt to the changes that we have made to the world". There is no better example than the gaining of weight.

It is important that you decide how much of a factor weight loss is going to be in your fitness program. But remember not to go by bodyweight alone. Muscle weighs more than fat so you can be losing fat but gaining weight.

Weight gain often comes gradually without our noticing it. My way of keeping track of my weight is my belt. I have the same belt that I have had for years and every time I put it on, I count with my finger how many holes there are to the last one. I use the second-to-last belt hole but can tighten to the last one without discomfort. That is right about where I want to be.

That is the trouble with getting new clothes particularly, for men, something like a belt that goes around the waist. It makes it more likely for us to gain weight without really realizing it.

I have a professional scale, but don't even weigh myself anymore. Bodyweight can be deceptive, primarily because water is a factor, especially if you don't always use the same scale. I just go by my belt.

The physical principle behind gaining or losing weight is simple. Fat is stored energy, and energy is measured in calories. Movement, or any activity of the body, expends energy. We require food to give us the energy to live and to move. If the food that we take in contains more energy than our bodies use, the excess energy is stored as fat. If our bodies use more energy than we take in with our food our bodies will burn fat, or other bodily tissues when the fat is gone, to make up the energy deficit.

As the goal of a fitness program, weight loss differs from the building of strength, endurance or, stamina in that all that matters is the amount of movement that the body does. It does not matter how easy or difficult the movement is. If the movement expends energy, as all movement does, it will contribute to weight loss. The way to increase strength, endurance or, stamina is to push the body toward it's limits in those areas, which necessarily involves difficulty. The way to lose weight is simply to do a lot of movement, and it doesn't really matter how easy or difficult that movement is.

In an average person, walking moderate distances will not do much to build strength or endurance or stamina. But it will contribute significantly to weight loss. All that matters in weight loss is how much mass is moved over how much distance, regardless of how easy or difficult it is.

With regard to the other aspects of physical fitness, strength, endurance and, stamina, activity for losing weight correlates most closely with training for stamina, second with endurance, and last with strength. That means that activities associated with building stamina, which is cardiovascular endurance, which is typically running, will tend to contribute to weight loss more than activities that build strength, typically weight-lifting.

The reason is that although weight-lifting is certainly moving mass, running or doing repetitive endurance exercises like pushups ends up moving more overall mass over more overall distance, and thus contributes more to weight loss.

This means that, in a fitness program with the emphasis on

weight loss there will be more total body movement, which may include such activities as walking, than there would be in training just for the other aspects of fitness. But this total body movement will not typically be as difficult as in training primarily for strength, endurance or, stamina, becasuse it is not really necessary to push the body to it's limits in order to lose weight.

In no way does this mean that training for the different aspects of fitness is completely separate. Strength or endurance training will tone the muscles. Tone is the tension in the muscles even when they are not being used. Tone itself uses up energy so that toned muscles use more energy even when the muscles are not being used, and that contributes to weight loss.

It is always advisable to work on the other aspects of fitness along with losing weight. Many people who have lost weight, but without building the body, have complained that they now feel "weak" and "flabby". One peril of doing all of the movement that it will take to lose weight is that it may make you hungry. If you reason that, "Well, I did my walk and my training so now I can afford to have a piece of cake", that may erase the gain that you have just made.

If you have too much weight, try to figure out why you gained that weight. That is part of the process of not gaining it back.

Weight loss usually involves both diet and exercise. But keep the two in perspective. If you are weak from hunger so that you can't properly do your exercise program, that isn't any good either.

9) INITIAL APPROACH TO FITNESS

All right, so you know that an exercise program would be a very good thing. So how do you begin?

If you haven't exercised in a long time, or ever, and do not do heavy physical work, do not just plunge into exercise. Your body needs time to adapt.

At the beginning of an exercise program, I think it is good to spend a couple of weeks or so doing some fairly easy exercises. Get used to the movements and to weaving an exercise routine into your life. See how it goes and where you stand with regard to physical fitness. You will soon feel how valuable it is and will want to do more. Then you can take it further.

This initial period of your exercise program should also be spent doing some more thinking about what exactly fitness means to you. What do you want to be, or to look, like or to be able to do when you are fit?

When I first decided that I had to start exercising, at age 15, I didn't have any set program. For a couple of weeks I just "messed around" with exercise, doing a few exercises that I was familiar with, mainly pushups. But that gave me a chance to get used to exercising, to decide what fitness meant to me, and to see where I stood, without the pressure of completing a required routine. Once I saw how beneficial exercise is, I became devoted to fitness from that day until now.

10) EXERCISES

With the internet today you can see just how exercises should be done. I just want to discuss a few basic exercises here and the muscle groups that they involve.

That old standby, pushups, are done by lying in a face down position, on the floor for men, and "pushing up" until the arms are straight. Women usually do pushups against an immovable object, such as a counter. These exercise the upper body, the pectoral (chest), shoulders and, triceps. But they do not work the biceps that much. The barbell equivalent of pushups is the bench press.

There is another possible exercise that uses approximately the same upper body muscles as pushups but requires, and thus builds, more strength because the feet are not on the floor. That exercise is dips but it requires some improvising unless you go to a gym. Dips are, as the name suggests, dipping the body down and bringing it back up. I have a dryer and a sink next to it in the basement. If I put a board across the sink, it will be at the same level as the dryer. I can support my body with one hand on the dryer and the other on the board, and then dip down by bending the arms and then back up. This is a strength-building exercise for the lower chest, the triceps and, the shoulders.

A variation of the pushup is one-armed pushups. As the name implies, the exercise is done with one arm, rather than with both hands on the floor. It may be required to lightly hold onto something, such as a chair, for support with the other hand. The difference between the two versions is that two-arm pushups, the motion being easier so that more repetitions can be done, is more of an endurance exercise. While one-arm pushups, in which only a few repetitions are usually possible, is more about building strength. Obviously, one-arm pushups must be done equally on both sides for balanced development.

Another pushup variation, which can be alternated with grip exercises, is fingertip pushups. This exercises the grip and forearm muscles.

Pressing weights overhead, whether dumbells or a barbell, exercises the shoulder muscles and triceps, the backs of the arms. The triceps are exercised by any motion that straightens the arms.

Pulling a weight down, or pulling the body up by doing pull-ups or chin-ups, exercises the back muscles, known as the laterals or "lats". As with pushups, pull-ups are using the body's weight as the resistance. The same back muscles are also exercised by lifting a weight up from the floor. Pulling the weight involves more the upper back and lifting it off the floor involves more the lower back.

The biceps, the inner arm muscles that pull the hands to the shoulders when starting from a straight-arm position, are exercised by "curling" a barbell or dumbell or by pull-ups (chin-ups).

The majority of the bulk of the upper arm is actually in the triceps, so-named because they have three components, not in the biceps, so-named because they have two components.

The forearm muscles are exercised by either closing the hands in a gripping movement or by pulling something, either backwards or forwards, with the hands while keeping the forearms stationary. Many people buy a simple grip exerciser or crumple a newspaper to squeeze.

The thigh muscles are exercised by doing knee bends, or squats, with or without a weight on the shoulders, or by pressing against some kind of weight with the feet.

The calf muscles are exercised by "calf raises", such as standing on a step with the toes and raising up by using the calves.

Doing one movement of an exercise, or a few repetitions that are near the maximum of your lifing ability, will build strength. Doing many repetitions of an exercise, to do the maximum number possible, will build endurance. Bench pressing is typically to build strength in the upper body, while pushups would be used to build endurance. It is strength training that builds the most muscle mass.

Stamina, which is cardio-vascular endurance, is built by

activities with a lot of movement in a short period of time, typically running.

Remember that weight loss, if it is a goal, requires a lot of movement but it doesn't so much matter how easy or difficult that movement is. What matters is the total amount of mass moved over the total distance.

When exercising to gain fitness for a particular sport, remember that the movements of the exercises should resemble the movements involved in the sport. If you were going to be a runner, and that was your primary objective, you probably wouldn't train for it by lifting heavy weights. Running is a fast movement and lifting heavy weights is necessarily a slow movement. Although you might do weight training to build strength in the sport's off-season.

11) SPECIAL BODY PARTS-THE NECK, STOMACH AND, LOWER BACK

There are three special areas that I would like to discuss.

The first is the neck. The muscles of the neck move the head. These muscles, which too often get ignored although the muscles in the neck do gain some benefit from other upper-body movements, require exercise too. The neck not only protects the breathing apparatus but also the spine. The primary benefit of strengthening the neck muscles, aside from keeping the development of the entire body in synch, is that it helps to prevent injury. Car accident injuries too often involve the neck because, if the body is restrained by the seatbelt and car comes to a very sudden stop, the head still has the forward momentum.

The neck muscles can be exercised in an isometric way, by pushing against the hands in a frontward motion, then backward, then to each side. My way of exercising the neck is simple. It is by not using a hair dryer.

The way to dry your hair is to shake the head vigorously, repeating several times a couple of minutes or so apart, until the hair is dry. Not only will your hair be dry, your neck muscles will have gotten a very good workout.

The second special area is the stomach. The stomach muscles, or abdominals, do not lift anything other than your body. The stomach muscles lift you up from a lying-down position. But no one would say that they are not very important. It is the stomach muscles that make you look trim and "in-shape". Trimming away fat and developing the stomach can even give the highly-prized "six-pack" "abs". When I was young, I went through an exercise phase when I was a "stomach fanatic".

Today I do two exercises for the stomach, although they do get some benefit from other exercises such as pushups and pull-ups. I do crunches, lying on an exercise bench, with the feet up and the body still, and raising the head repeatedly so that it tenses the abdominal muscles. I also do twists, standing upright and twisting vigorously from left to right, keeping the hips nearly still, with the arms extended so that the right hand touches the left shoulder and vice-versa. Crunches exercise the muscles on the front of the abdominals and twists the muscles on the sides. We will get to your actual exercises later.

Since those twists involve quite a bit of total movement, that makes them good for losing weight, and they tone the midsection at the same time. Another old weight-loss standby, and one that gives the entire body some exercise especially the calf muscles, is jumping jacks. But jumping jacks probably cannot be done in an apartment unless you are on the ground floor.

Well-developed abdominal muscles not only benefit the body's appearance and enable it to move faster, they also improve the reflexes. A person with a taut stomach generally has better reflexes, as most athletes are aware.

The third muscle group that deserves special consideration is the lower back. This is an area that sometimes sustains injury. The muscles of the lower back come into play when something is lifted off the floor. The age-old advice when lifting is to "bend your knees, not your back". Many exercise programs actually miss the muscles of the lower back.

The best thing to do is to get an object with some weight, such as a storage bin or small trunk. Lift it to a standing straight up position for about five repetitions, several times per week. This will keep the muscles of the lower back strong. You do not have to do this if you are lifting weights in a way that involves the lower back. Also, lifting anything with a smooth and steady movement keeps it from injury, although a lower back injury is usually only a pulled muscle that gets better in a few days.

12) BREATHING

How often do you think about your breathing? It is actually the most important thing that your body does. Oxygen is even more important than water and food.

We know that breathing is important in physical fitness. The definition of stamina is how well the heart and lungs can provide the increased oxygen that is necessary for the muscles during exertion. When doing any sudden physical thrust or movement, including shooting a gun, it should be done when exhaling and not when inhaling.

But did you know that few people use their full lung capacity during ordinary breathing?

While sitting or standing, without any exertion, where is the expansion of your abdomen taking place when you inhale?

If the primary expansion is in your chest, that means that you are not utilizing your full lung capacity. The primary expansion should be your stomach.

Fortunately, we can exercise the breathing to attain full lung capacity.

While sitting down without any exertion, fill your lungs as full as you can. Hold it for about ten seconds and then exhale as fully as you can. Repeat this simple exercise ten times and then every day. Breathe very deeply, as deeply as you can. Before long, your ordinary breathing should have the primary expansion in the stomach. The exercises can then be discontinued.

REVERSE EXERCISES

Here is something worth considering. It is a way to quickly build strength and is done by simply reversing the exercise. This can be done with either calisthenics or weights.

Consider ordinary pushups. I like to reference pushups because it is a simple exercise that just about everyone would be familiar with. To reverse them, start at the top of the exercise position with the arms fully extended and the body at it's highest position off the floor.

Begin by lowering the body, as you usually would, but lower it very, very, very slowly, so that it takes close to a full minute to reach the bottom of the exercise. Then, raise the body up quickly and begin the very slow lowering process again. This puts the work on the negative, the lowering side, of the exercise.

Reverse exercising can also be done with knee bends, and with some barbell exercises such as curls.

To do a reverse exercise for the stomach, this is difficult, lie down on some kind of mat. Hold onto something that is just above your head. Put the feet together and the legs straight. Raise the legs to an angle of about 45 degrees. Then, lower the legs doen to the mat very, very, very slowly.

The number of repetitions that can be done exercising like this will be low, maybe around five. While it is strengthening, it may not be very good for endurance. Reverse exercising is somewhat of a fad, but there are a few people who claim to have gotten outstanding results with it.

MY MOTHER

Let me just tell you the story of my late mother, when she was in her 80s. She provided one of the best lessons that I have seen about the value of exercise, particularly to the elderly.

She spent some time in hospital and in rehabilitation afterward, where she was given some exercises to do. She didn't have a lot of enthusiasm for exercise but I tried to convince her of it's value. When my mother did her exercise program, and when she didn't, she was like two different people.

When she was doing the exercises every day, she would come shopping and walk around the store with no problem, and often ask to be taken to another store afterward. But when she wasn't doing the exercises, she could barely make it around the store and had to keep resting.

She fell down several times, always when she wasn't doing the exercises. Falling would convince her how important exercise was and she would go back to the program, at least for a while. This convinced me more than ever before of the importance of an exercise program, and that it should be a life-long endeavor. If there was a pill that could have made the difference in my mother from when she was exercising to when she wasn't, it would surely have been the greatest invention the world has ever seen.

MILO OF CROTON

Have you ever wondered how the idea of building strength and fitness by progressive resistance training began?

From ancient Greece comes the story of Milo of Croton. He got the idea that, if he could carry a newborn calf and then carry it every day, his body would become stronger as the calf grew bigger and heavier and, when the calf was fully grown, he would still be able to carry it.

A SUBSTITUTE FOR RUNNING

I know that running is a very valuable exercise. But I am not a runner. The reason is that it takes too much time and then you still have to exercise the upper body. It would be good to alternate running with exercises, running one day and exercise the next, and that is what some people do. Or running when it's sunny and exercising indoors when it's raining.

But I have always sought a substitute for running, and the stamina that it provides. I thought of high-count pushups as "running with the arms instead of the legs". The set would elevate my heart rate and breathing, as if I had sprinted, but it would work the upper body as well.

One possible substitute for running, but done indoors and working the upper body at the same time, is a "rolling stamina" series of exercises. The stamina that running provides is the endurance of the cardio-vascular system, the heart and lungs, as they provide oxygen to the muscles. It does not matter to the heart and lungs where the muscles undergoing the exertion are, the legs or the upper body. It will build stamina just the same.

An example of a "rolling stamina" series of exercises is to do as many pushups as possible. That will elevate the heart and lungs rate but the endurance of the muscles of the upper body limit how many pushups can be done. Immediately, or almost immediately, after completing the set of pushups do a set of knee bends. This will keep the heart and lung rate elevated but by using a different set of muscles than the already-tired upper body after the pushups.

Next add another exercise that will keep the rate of the heart and lungs going, maybe doing some more pushups. Then maybe a few more knee bands. The objective of this "rolling stamina" sequence is to get the cardio-vascular stamina benefit of running and exercising the rest of the body as well.

USING YOUR OWN BODYWEIGHT

There is an advantage to being heavy. It makes it easier to

build strength by calisthenics, using your own bodyweight. Calisthenics like pushups and pull-ups (chin-ups) work by making use of your own bodyweight as resistance. If you are heavy, part of your objective may be to lose weight. But in the meantime being heavier will mean being able to do fewer repetitions of an exercise, which means it will build less endurance, but the additional weight will build more strength. Dips, as described above, is an especially good strength building exercise for the upper body if the trainee is heavier.

MAKE A WORKOUT OUT OF IT

Your workout may not be the only place for you to get valuable exercise. When you do a physical task that requires some exertion there may be ways to "make a workout out of it". The main thing to be concerned about is making sure that you give both sides of the body equal work.

An ideal example is shoveling snow in the winter. Most people that are right-handed will hold the handle of the shovel with their left hand and hold the body of the shovel with their right hand. This means pushing with the left hand and pulling with the right hand. But that develops the body unequally. To "make a workout out of it", you should alternate sides periodically.

If you carry something heavy with one hand, such as a container of water, try to carry it more with your weak side to help to be sure that side keeps up with your stronger side.

"Making a workout out of it" does not mean you shouldn't do your regular workout. But when doing physical tasks requiring exertion, a little creativity may make it possible to add to the benefits of the regular workout.

CHAPTER THREE

THE PSYCHOLOGY OF EXERCISE

1) NEGATIVES

Plenty of people have a negative concept of exercise in some way, and we want to make sure that any such thing does not hold you back. Maybe it was from school, the exercises required in gym class. Maybe it was from the military using exercise as punishment. Maybe one of your siblings was the "athlete" of the family while you had some other role, and exercise is not in your domain.

Being pressured to excel in sports by parents with visions of their son or daughter as a superstar athlete probably doesn't help. "Hockey dads" are particularly notorious.

There is still some negative stereotypes about people who exercise. I recall a television show where someone was described as "He looks like he could lift a car but wouldn't be able to spell it".

We are used to trying to make physical work as easy as possible. We cannot do this with exercise, since it would defeat the very purpose of it. But it is true that in exercising, we want to work "smart" as well as working hard.

Some people do not want to be fit and healthy. I recall one person who was physically infirm. I noticed a number of things that she could do to improve her health, but then saw clearly that she wasn't interested. She had people around her who coddled and sympathized with her, and she liked it that way.

We still have not completely realized the need for exercise. In days past, people didn't live as long and most engaged in physical labor. Modern medicine has gotten people living longer but technology has taken away the majority of the physical work. Our bodies were not intended to be sedentary and it is causing all manner of health problems. Once again, if I had to describe our era in one sentence it would be "We have reached the point where we can change the world faster than we can adapt to the changes that we have made in the world".

One adaptation that we have got to make is to exercise.

One issue with exercise is that videos and guides to it tend to be written by athletes, to whom working out is the most important thing in life. The other major source of instruction is the medical field, with exercises for medical ailments.

This book is aimed at everyone else. Exercise is not the

most important thing in my life. I have a religion, I am a Christian. I also have intellectual work for my writing. I consider both of these as more important than exercise. Of the mind, the body and, the spirit, I actually consider the body as the least important.

But yet it is important, and we have to take care of it. You have far more control over your health and fitness than you probably realize. What I want here is for your health and fitness to be the best it possibly can, but without displacing everything else in your life. I am sure that we can accomplish just that. Just the fact that you have read this far shows that you have the motivation to take charge of your health and fitness.

2) PSYCHOLOGICAL TRICKS

All of the people who keep up a successful exercise program over the long term have one thing in common. They all have psychological tricks that get them through their workouts. I have a whole repertoire of psychological tricks that I have used to get the most out of exercise.

First, at least in the beginning, write down the exercise program that you are going to do. Not only will this keep track of the exercises, it will make you feel obligated to complete the schedule. But don't write down a schedule that is so ambitious that you are not going to do it for long.

Suppose that you are doing an endurance exercise and want to do the maximum number that you can do. You are sure that you can do 50 pushups but want to try to do more. DO NOT count from 1 to 50 as you are doing the repetitions of the exercise. Count to 30 and than start the count over. See if you can "trick" your body into doing a few more repetitions because it "thinks" it hasn't done 50 yet.

If you are doing a repetitive exercise, think about how easy it is during the early repetitions. "This is a piece of cake".

One of the worst words in the dictionary is "talent". Erase this word from your vocabulary. Athletes, and anyone else, who are "talented" are not talented. They just keep on trying and improving. Then someone without the same sense of improvement will say "Oh, that person is so talented". Even when someone seems to be an "instant success" at something, it is probable that they have been doing some other activity which involves similar patterns.

The way you feel before you workout, barring illness, actually has little to do with how your workout will go. Many times I have not felt like exercising, but have done it anyway, and it has gone really well. If you don't feel like exercising, but you do have time and there is no real reason why you shouldn't be doing it, then just start doing it. Once you get into exercise your attitude will change.

Another psychological trick is bright colors. The plates that go on barbells, for one example, are often painted in bright colors. This makes the weights seem "friendly". If you go into a gym and the weights look like raw iron, they seem to say "Look at how heavy I am. I am made of iron. You could not possibly lift me so just get out of the gym and go back home". But if the weights are painted yellow, blue and, green, they look like a meadow on a sunny day. The weights are your friends, there to help you get fit. Even though they weigh exactly the same as the ones that look like raw iron, they somehow seem easier to lift.

Negatives can also be motivating. Discipline is necessary for an exercise program and many people have a built in guilt complex about exercise, if they know that they could have and should have exercised today, but didn't.

There is the old strategy of music. Get a song that you really like, that puts energy into you. But then don't listen to it. Save it for when you are trying to accomplish an athletic feat. When I used to listen to music, "Gimme Shelter" was my song. It was helpful that it was a long song.

Don't think this is silly because it isn't. Your body is controlled by your mind. Succeeding at athletics or exercise is usually not about being a "Superman" or "Superwoman". It is about gathering up all of the little advantages that you can get, both physical and psychological, and putting them all together.

3) "LETS MAKE SOME NEW FRIENDS"

Let me introduce you to a few new friends. As you progress in exercise you will become familiar with them. In fact, they have become friends with every great athlete who has ever lived.

These are the kind of friends that you may not like at first. But as you progress you will see how much they are really there to help you.

Your first new friend is tiredness. When you use your muscles they will get tired. That is because the muscles secrete lactic acid when they are used, and this lactic acid builds up. When you rest your blood circulation drains it away. When you do aerobic exercise your heart will be beating faster and you will be breathing more heavily. At some point, you will have to rest until it returns to normal.

But this means that your exercise session is working. You are pushing your body toward it's physical limits and that is what you want to do. Your physical limits will adjust accordingly and you will gradually be able to do more and more. That is the purpose of exercise. If you exercise and are not tired at all that means that your exercise really isn't doing a lot of good. Depending on what your exercise goals are, you should be pushing your strength, endurance and, stamina to near their limits several times a week.

Your next new friend is soreness. When you exercise and then the muscles are sore the next day, that is the muscles telling you that they need more time to recover before you do those exercises again.

But, once again, that means that your exercises are achieving their desired effect. Remember how building up the muscles works. Exercise actually tears down the muscles. but then your body builds them back up. In order to adjust to the demand that exercise is putting on your body not only does your body build the muscles back up, it builds them so that they are a little bit stronger and better than before. That is the whole principle of exercise. When the muscles that you have exercised are sore the next day, thet means your body is in the process of building them back up, to be more capable than before, and needs a little bit more time.

You can "work around" soreness. If your legs are sore, you can still exercise your upper body, and vice versa.

Another new friend is hunger. Again, it is the kind of friend that you may not like at first. But your muscles are composed largely of protein. When you have exercised and then are hungrier than usual the next day, that means that your exercise session was a success because your body is asking for more protein so that it can strengthen itself.

If losing weight is part of your fitness goal then hunger is a friend in another way. It means that your body would like more food than it is getting, and until it gets more food it is using the fat stored in your body for food. That means you are losing weight.

People who are successful at their fitness or athletic program, and make exercise a lifelong habit, all have found a way to "make friends" with tiredness, soreness and, hunger, by remembering that they are really signs of progress.

It is not all "new friends" that you will be making. There is also an enemy. The name of this enemy is "The Law of Diminishing Returns". But you can avoid having your progress hindered by The Law of Diminishing Returns, if you follow a simple strategy.

Unlike tiredness and soreness, The Law of Diminishing Returns applies to both diet and exercise. You may have a good diet but if you keep eating the same foods all the time your body will have an abundance of the nutrients in those foods, which is a good thing. But since no single set of foods has all of the nutrients that you need, "The Law of Diminshing Returns will set in. That means that you will be getting less benefit from your diet than you were when you got on a good diet to begin with.

The Law of Diminishing Returns, with regard to diet, can be defeated by keeping the staple foods, as discussed earlier, and then varying the rest by the week.

The Law of Diminishing Returns will try to hinder your progress in exercise as well. As discussed earlier if you keep doing the same exercises in the same way, while that is certainly better than nothing, it is exercising the muscles from the same angle all the time. The body will adjust to this demand, but then progress will level off.

The way to defeat the Law of Diminishing Returns, with regard to exercise, is to vary the exercises. You might switch up your exercises program perdically, maybe keeping a few "staple" exercises, but changing the exercises done for different muscle groups. When you do the same exercises, you can put some variety in by changing the width of your grip with some exercises. If lifting weights, you can alternate doing fewer repetitions with a heavier weight with doing more repetitions with a lighter weight.

When dealing with diet or exercise, always "keep an eye" on The Law of Dimishing Returns. You do not have to let it hinder your progress.

4) EXERCISE AS AN OUTLET

One of the things that is absolutely wonderful about exercise is how well it works as a drain for stress. I was in an accident once and couldn't exercise for about six weeks. Before long, I noticed that I wasn't handling everyday stress as well as I was before. But after I could get back into my exercise program, everything was soon back to normal.

A wonderful thing to be able to do is to gather all of the stresses and frustrations that go with life and, instead of getting angry or upset about them, put their energy into your workout. Whenever you are treated unfairly, just use it to motivate you to do a better workout than ever.

Too often, people cope with stress in destructive ways. Your exercise program will give you a chance to do it in a very constructive way.

5) EXERCISE AS A LOT OF FUN

Here is something that is as important as anything to do with exercise and will likely determine if your program will be a success or failure. It is really simple but extremely important. Always think of exercise as fun. Never think of exercise as work or you will never get the most out of it. It is absolutely imperative that you think of exercise as fun.

If you are asked why you exercise the best answer is because you are having fun. Of course you want to be fit too, but the primary reason is that it is so much fun. Your body was designed and intended to be active and you enjoy exercise so much because it is fulfilling that intent.

But what makes exercise even more fun is all that you are gaining from it. I have never heard of anyone who regretted exercise. Why do you think so many people struggle in gyms? Because it is worth it, that's why. It is more than worth it. One of the greatest things in life is as simple as exercise. Those who don't exercise either do not realize how valuable it is or have not managed to weave it into their lives. If anyone could invent a pill that could give you all of the benefits os a sensible exercise program, it would certainly be the greatest invention in history.

6) ATTACH EXERCISE TO MOTIVATION

Find a way to attach your exercise program to something that inspires or motivates you. It doesn't have to make sense, all it has to do is to get you through a productive workout.

Here is my story. After I had completed high school in the U.S. I went to visit my native England. I didn't have a job there, I had finished high school, and wasn't yet religious. This cleared the way for exercise, which I had been doing for some time, to be my primary concern.

I didn't have any exercise equipment but every morning before going out I would do exercises like pushups, and others that I could do without any equipment. In my first set of pushups each morning I would strive to do the maximum number possible. Every day I would set a goal of how many I would do the following morning, and then put everything into trying to meet that goal.

What happened is, from that point on, the place where I was born reminded me of exercise. One morning there I had done more pushups, in a single set, than I had ever done before. Afterward, I waited in a brick bus shelter for the bus to go into town. I was thinking of all the possibilities that I might be able to accomplish. If ever there is a morning when I don't feel like exercising, all I have to do is get on Google Street View and visit that bus stop. Even a light drizzly rain immediately puts me in the frame of mind to get into my exercise program.

Running or exercising outside has long been a way to connect with nature. Not only are you enjoying the outside but you are getting your body away from being sedentary and restoring it to it's naturally active state.

For some people, exercise is a way to reconnect with their youth. For about an hour, four times a week, I treat my body like it was 18 or 19 again, and my body seems to really enjoy exercising along Memory Lane.

I read about one man who was an athlete in his youth. At the same time, he had a really cool car. What he did to help motivate him to get back into exercise was to get metal weights and paint them, with automotive paint, the same color that his car had been.

The wonderful thing about attaching your exercise program to something that motivates or inspires you is that it doesn't have to make any sense. All it has to do is to get you to put your best into your exercise program.

If you like knights and castles then putting a picture of a castle where you exercise will remind you that you have to be in shape to be a modern-day knight.

What about patriotism? If you are healthy and in-shape, you will likely be less of a burden on your country's health care system. And it is a credit to any ethnic group or country to have it's citizens strong and fit and healthy.

You have heard of success gurus exhorting people to "dress

for success". What about exercise? The outfit that you wear during your program can be very useful in reminding you that you have to "live up" to the way you are dressed. If you are dressed like a good athlete then that might convince your body to perform accordingly. Associating exercise with the bright colors of a soccer (football) outfit might be helpful.

Seeking sports proficiency can be the best motivation to exercise. Competition sometimes brings out the worst in people, but it can also bring out the best. Fitness is an important factor, often the most important factor, in any sport. Training for sports is usually split between exercises that are beneficial to the sport, and then playing the sport itself.

When a person is healthy and fit they inevitably look better than they would otherwise. What better motivation to exercise and get on the best possible diet is there than this?

Do women ever stop to think that a diet with emphasis on vegetables in general, and carrots in particular, might be able to put the beauty industry out of business? It is virtually impossible to have a lot of vegetables every day, especially carrots, without being physically attractive.

A powerful source of motivation to exercise is to see how other people are motivated. If all of these people are putting so much into their exercise than it must really be worthwhile. You may also get valuable information and see how their programs are working.

7) BE RESOURCEFUL

In your diet, and especially your exercise program, always be looking for ways to get done what needs to be done and to continuously improve. Be resourceful. There is always a better way to do things. Keep looking for ways to improve and you will be delighted with the progress that you make. I am a writer and a lot of my writing is about science. This is where I got my scientific way of thinking from, always looking for more efficiency and ways to improve my exercise program. It was like a laboratory.

CHAPTER FOUR

GETTING STARTED

1) TAKE CHARGE

You must really want to be the best that you can be in health and fitness or you wouldn't have read this far. It's time to take charge of your health and fitness. It is your responsibility and it is a lot more under your control than you probably realize.

No matter how many CAT scans, X-rays and, MRIs you have done, no matter how many doctors you see, none of those have what you have. You are the only one that is actually inside your body. You can sense what is going on inside your body like nothing else can, and now we are going to make the most out of that advantage. We are going to put what we have learned into practice.

2) EVERYONE IS DIFFERENT

What everyone needs to keep in mind about exercise programs and diets is that everyone is different. What works for one person may not work as well, or may work better, for another. That is why, to be at your peak of health and fitness, you must keep learning, and applying what you have learned, and improving.

Suppose, again, that you study auto mechanics. You will learn all about how cars work, how and why they break down, and how to repair tham when they do. But what has to be taken into account is that every car is different. Each make and model of car has it's own quirks and strengths and weaknesses. Human bodies, as well as minds, are exactly the same way.

There are a million diets and exercise programs online and in books. But these are general programs, or programs that worked well for someone else. That is not to say that they wouldn't work for you but to be absolutely at your best you have to keep analyzing and improving until you get the diet and exercise program that is absolutely the best for you. Exactly what you want out of fitness may not be the same as for anyone else. the exercise program that you are most likely to stay with is one that you develop yourself. But the thing that you always have going for you in the meantime is that virtually any exercise program is better than doing nothing.

3) SIMPLE HEALTH SOLUTIONS

I am certainly not telling you that it will never be necessary to see a doctor. But there are so many minor health issues that have a simple solution waiting to be found. Here are a few of mine.

For years I suffered from dry skin, particularly in the winter because the air from the furnace is dry. I would put lotions on the areas that would be dry at night, but it wouldn't completely solve it. I would keep a bowl of water in my bedroom and the room where I would spend most of my time, but it still didn't completely solve it.

As it turned out, there was a very simple solution that I happened across. When I was boiling water for a meal, I would put a lid on the pot so that it would boil faster. One day I got the idea that if I would leave the lid off the pot, the steam would put enough humidity into the air that it would solve my dry skin. It worked wonders and I do not have the slightest dry skin any more.

Sometimes my eyes would be dry. All they needed was a little bit more moisture. Ordinary eye drops once a day solved the problem.

Really the only health issues I have had have been dental. But I found something out and, at this point, I haven't had to see a dentist in several years. Brushing the teeth once a day isn't enough. Food residue begins to decay the teeth after about 12 hours. Thoroughly cleaning the teeth twice a day is necessary. An apple as the last thing you eat every day also helps to clean the teeth.

If you can't sleep, just relax. Relaxing is almost as restful as sleeping.

I have reduced the number of times that I get the flu. When it is flu season, and you feel that you have been exposed to it, drink a lot of water for the rest of the day. It is all right to skip exercise that day but really drink a lot of water, far more than you usually do. That should stop the flu from catching on to your system. If you have been exposed to the flu, but it hasn't caught on in your system, that means that you should be immune to that strain of the flu. But there may be another strain later on in the winter and you have to get immunity to that one too. I have never gotten a flu shot but this is the same principle.

The old advice about washing your hands is right. When it is flu season, often wash your hands and do not unnecessarily touch your face with your hands.

When standing for most of the day, I would sometimes get tension in my back. As it turned out, there was a stretching exercise that I had forgotten about. Lying on a mattress, with the body more toward the lower end of the mattress than usual, throwing the feet over the head, and holding the position for about twenty seconds, solved the problem. My back just needed some stretching from a different angle, and the tension went away immediately.

4) IMPROVISE

Get that attitude of improvising and adapting. Find a way to work around whatever situations and shortcomings arise. There is always a way to do it.

One man who used to exercise at a gym, but had a hectic schedule, came up with the idea of always keeping his gym bag in his car. If the opportunity arose, he could stop at the gym for an hour or so.

You are in charge of your health and fitness now and you are going to make the very best of it. Most of the advice out there is good advice, but is general advice. You are unique, not exactly like anyone else in either body of what you want from fitness, and you are going to set about zeroing in on the diet and exercise routine that is exactly right for you and what you want to be. What you have here is enough to get you moving in the right direction.

Once you get going in your fitness program, you may make up your own exercises. People who are always traveling have come up with ingenious ways to use their luggage to do exercises, as well as calisthenics like pushups, twists and, knee bends that can be done anywhere. Just remember the two principles that you have to exercise the entire body and take the muscles through their full range of motion.

One man who had a swimming pool got two pieces of plywood, attached a handle near the end of each piece, then attached a brace to each piece that his forearm would fit through it as he held onto the handles. The result was like a pair of "wings" with which he could exercise displacing water by pushing forward, which exercised the front muscles such as the chest, and then pushing back, to exercise the back muscles and the back of the shoulders. It took some trial and error to get it just right.

Maybe your local store has something that might be useful for exercise. What about a container of cat litter with a handle?

Another man came up with the simple idea of pushing his car for one of his exercises, up a slight incline.

If you are fortunate enough to live near a steep hill, just a walk up the hill is likely as good as running on flat ground.

Likewise, if you live on the sixth floor you should still do an exercise session but it will work wonders to always take the stairs up. If I lived on a sixth floor you would never see me going up in the elevator.

I came up with the idea of jumping as an exercise, in seeking a replacement for running. Just put a stick or piece of tape at a comfortable height from the floor and then start jumping over it, back and forth, doing about 20 repetitions. Obviously this cannot be done if you live in an apartment building, but you can find something else to replace it.

5) LET'S GET STARTED

All right, let's get started. From this point on it's all up to you. Begin with these simple exercises here for maybe a couple of weeks. This will get you used to exercising and making it part of your life. Decide when during the day you will have the best opportunity to exercise. Evaluate where you stand with regard to fitness. If you get a little bit sore, that means the exercise is working and needs a little more time to recuperate before you continue the exercise.

This doesn't matter who you are, male or female, young or old. All the while be thinking what fitness means to you, what you want to be and what you want from it. When the initial period of two weeks or so are over, you can continue doing these exercises and also begin to add more. When you begin to see how wonderful fitness is, you will want to do more. You can begin your program in your ordinary clothes but will probably want to get an appropriate exercise outfit soon. Keep these three calisthenic exercises here in mind because they are quick and easy to do if something arises and you don't have time to do your regular exercise routine.

Try pushups, in some form, this will strengthen, and enable you to evaluate, your upper body. This is the first thing I did when I just got tired of feeling out of shape and decided that I had to start exercising.

If you are male, try pushups on the floor. You can start with a few, maybe 5-10. Keep your back straight. Maybe you can look online to see an illustration of how they are done.

If you are female, or too heavy to do pushups on the floor, then lean against a sink or other counter. Put all of your energy into it because you are beginning a wonderful new journey.

Next, let's do some twists. This will strengthen the entire midsection. Stand with your feet about shoulder width apart. Extend both arms in front of you. Now twist vigorously to your right so that your left hand touches near your right shoulder. Now repeat so that your right hand touches near your left shoulder. Don't just go through the motions, put a lot of energy into it. To begin with, do at least 30 repetitions.

Twisting like this involves quite a bit of motion. That means that this exercise will ge useful in losing weight, if that is one of your goals. Remember that weight gain or loss obeys the laws of physics. It doesn't so much matter how easy or difficult the motion is, just the total amount of movement that is done.

The third, and final, exercise that we will start with are knee bends. Stand comfortably and then bend your knees all the way down and then back up. At the bottom of the exercise the tops of your thighs should be parallel to the floor. Hold onto something, to begin with, if you have to. Make sure to bend all the way down and bend your knees and not your back. this is a very beneficial exercise, some people just call them squats. Just start with a few repetitions and then see if your legs are sore tomorrow. if not, then continue nearly every day.

Also don't forget your breathing exercises, described earlier, to make sure that you are using your full lung capacity. These can be discontinued, as described earlier, when the goal is accomplished and the primary expansion during breathing is in the stomach rather than the chest. But these exercises do not necessarily have to be done at the same time as your beginning exercises described here.

Another exercise, remembering that the lower back is a critical area and that a lot of exercise routines actually miss it as described earlier, is to get a moderately heavy box, or other object, or small trunk, and lift it nearly daily for five repetitions or so. That will condition the muscles of the lower back, and make them much less susceptible to injury.

Depending on your present fitness level, if weight-loss is one of your goals, and you have a basement or live on a ground floor, you may want to include jumping jacks, as they involve a lot of total motion and are an old weight-loss standby exercise.

Finally, I asked God to give me good health.